DYNAMIC DIET

A Dietary Guide and Workbook
for Patients with

Irritable Bowel Syndrome

How to create *your diet*

to manage *your IBS*

Authors:

Dr. Ashkan Farhadi, MD, FACG
Gastroenterologist

Kelly Wyckoff, MS, RD, CNSD
Clinical Dietitian

SanitizAir, Inc.

ISBN: 1440471827
EAN: 9781440471827

Printed in the United States of America

Sales and Distribution
United States

Create Space Publishing

WWW. CREATESPACE.COM

Amazon.com

Note: The authors have made every effort to ensure that all the information and recommendations contained in this book are up to date and in accordance with the best knowledge available at the time of publication. However, since research and regulations constantly change clinical standards, the reader is urged to check this book's recommendations with a physician. The reader is cautioned that the purpose of this book is to inform and enlighten; the information contained herein is not intended as, and should not be employed as, a substitute for individual diagnosis and treatment by a competent health professional.

Table of Contents

The Role of Food in Health and Disease

Since ancient times, people have used nutritional management to treat common ailments. For many years, diet modification has been considered one of the major modalities in the treatment of a wide spectrum of ailments ranging from ordinary problems such as the common cold and fevers to serious illnesses such as cancers, infectious diseases and psychiatric illnesses.

The GI tract is the organ that directly interact with food by digesting and absorbing nutrients. It is widely accepted that strict diet adherence for the management of gastrointestinal disorders is of utmost importance. However, a review of the medical literature shows that most of these beliefs are mainly based on cultural values, personal experiences, and/or common sense, rather than on scientific research. Thus, overemphasis of these untested restrictions, which is a common practice by many health professionals and doctors, could result in unnecessary limitations of patients nutritional choices without any proven benefit. This is particularly true in patients with irritable bowel syndrome (IBS) in whom the disease symptoms, in some shape or form, correlate with the dietary profile.

Despite our growing understanding of the nature of IBS, our knowledge of the effect of nutritional factors in the pathogenesis of IBS is still rudimentary. Thus, it is not surprising that the best method of dietary management in IBS is based on symptom-oriented diet modification.

Overall, diet modification for patients with IBS is an important part in the management of IBS and should be viewed as a valuable tool to be used in combination with other strategies such as lifestyle changes, behavioral therapy, and pharmacologic treatment.

This handout and workbook are designed to improve your overall knowledge about various aspects of your diet and to help you explore your dietary choices to build your own diet that best suits your condition. This commonsense approach could be one of the most useful and least restrictive diet modifications you may select to manage your IBS.

How to Choose Your Diet

As mentioned above, choosing the right diet is an important tool for managing IBS. The main question is "How should you choose your diet?" There are several sources you can use to choose the appropriate diet:

1) Research
2) Allergy testing
3) Common knowledge
4) Others' experience
5) Personal experience

Research

There are several studies in which researchers have attempted to correlate diet intake with symptoms in patients with IBS. Subjects were asked to fill out a detailed questionnaire regarding their daily diet and symptoms. The results of these studies showed a large variability in each individual's food triggers. It also helped to provide a list of safe foods as well as common stimulant foods. However, a stimulant food for one individual could be a non-stimulant for another individual and vice versa.

Knowledge of this information will be helpful in guiding you to find your own stimulant and non-stimulant foods but would not serve as a dietary model. Some of the common stimulants include high-fat foods, cow's milk, yeast, egg whites, sorbitol, fructose, caffeine, and alcohol.

Fat is the single greatest GI stimulant, and high-fat meals may exacerbate symptoms. Fructose-restricted diets have been shown to reduce symptoms of IBS in some studies. Sorbitol, a sugar alcohol used in sugar-free products, may increase symptoms of gas, bloating and diarrhea when consumed in large quantities. In addition, caffeinated beverages and alcohol may stimulate the intestine and cause or exacerbate already existing diarrhea. On the other hand, potatoes, grapefruit, apricots, apples, barley, and lemons are among those food items with least amount of symptom exacerbation.

Allergy testing

There are a few studies that attempted to eliminate foods that produced an allergic reaction in either blood tests or skin allergy tests. Using skin allergy testing, one study found that 25% of a sample of individuals with IBS had a positive allergy test to a specific food. Despite some preliminary promising result with this strategy, these studies have not proved that allergy testing for specific food is a useful test that needs to be performed in all IBS patients for the purpose of food selection. These tests could be expensive, cumbersome, and in a significant number of cases, falsely positive. This may result in unnecessary restriction in dietary selection in large number of patients. Until improvement in the method of testing and further positive studies, this method is not recommended as part of the standard of care in individuals with IBS.

Common knowledge

Information from resources that can be considered common knowledge, such as the internet and books or other printed materials, could also be considered valuable; however, it would be hard to separate the baseless claims from the scientific and useful information. Thus, I encourage you to approach advice regarding changes in diet and dietary supplements with caution. I also encourage you to use your common sense in the decision-making process. As you know, several diet modifications for the management of IBS exist in the literature. Some of these measures even claim that they can completely cure this ailment. The following list addresses some of the common dietary advice that you have most likely encountered and provides recommendations about each one.

1. **Consume small, frequent meals (4 to 6 meals per day)**

   Rationale: It is important to eat small, frequent meals to ensure adequate calorie intake and to decrease the risk of developing cramps, diarrhea, and other symptoms that may occur with the consumption of large meals.

   Recommendation: This is an example of a widely accepted belief that more frequent but smaller meal portions could be helpful in IBS. There are no data to support this claim. This strategy may be helpful to a select group of subjects with

IBS who have a very sensitive GI tract and experience symptoms with larger meals. Our recommendation is that individuals base their decisions on personal experience and determine the amount of food that can be safely handled by their own digestive tract. In general, we suggest consuming three meals per day and avoiding erratic meal schedules, including skipping meals, to prevent disturbances in gastrointestinal physiological response.

2. **Dine on time**

   Rationale: It is important not to skip meals and to try to eat at roughly the same time each day to help regulate your bowel function.

   Recommendation: All of the physiological processes in the body are connected to our body's internal clock, and food digestion is not an exception. Thus, the function of most of our digestive hormones is affected by the time of day, and it is the best to use the system on its prime time. Having said that, there are no data to back the claim that erratic eating behavior is more prevalent in IBS subjects or that it could result in IBS or an IBS flare-up.

3. **Avoid spicy meals, salad dressing, red meat, and caffeine**

   Rationale: These food items are stimulants and contribute to GI symptoms.

   Recommendation: Based on our observations, stimulant foods are individualized and there is no predetermined list that fits everyone. Please refer to "the Dynamic Diet" section for a detailed discussion on this issue.

4. **Drink plenty of fluids**

   Rationale: Water is best to consume. Your body as well as your digestive tract lives in water and you should provide adequate hydration for your body.

   Recommendation: This is another non-evidence based piece of common advice for IBS patients. Drinking plenty of water during meals may increase your stomach size and cause dyspepsia and discomfort after the meal. We recommend consuming water as your body asks for it through your thirst cues.

5. **Do not eat on the run**

   Rationale: When eating on the run, it is easy to consume food too quickly and in larger amounts than you would normally eat when taking your time. In addition, eating on the run can also be very stressful, which can cause unwanted GI symptoms.

   Recommendation: Although this seems to be commonsense advice, there are no data to back it up. We recommend eating the way that is best for you, on the run or not on the run.

6. **Avoid distractions at meal times**

   Rationale: When dining with too much stimulation around you, mealtime can become stressful. Turn off the television and turn on calming music while you eat to reduce these stressors.

Recommendation: Eat as you like, with or without TV. Listen to your gut. Your symptoms will tell you to eat alone or in a big crowd, in silence or with loud music, or with or without TV.

7. **Dine out with caution**

   Rationale: Restaurant food may contain unknown ingredients or much more fat than homemade food, and the portion sizes may be larger than those we normally eat. All of these combined may cause unwanted GI symptoms.

   Recommendation: This is useful commonsense advice. When you choose to dine out, pay attention to the following:

   o Ensure that there are no surprise ingredients in what you order.

   o Consider that the portions in restaurants are typically much bigger. Request a box for the uneaten portion of the meal.

   o Ask for low-fat options.

Others' Experience

We recommend treating this similarly to general resources on the internet and in print. You should do your homework and create a diet that best suits you. Always take this advice and information with a grain of salt.

Personal Experience

Listen to your gut. This recommendation can provide you with the most reliable, practical and enforceable diet modification. But what does this really mean? It means that, through trial and error, you are in charge of creating your diet and excluding the diet elements that trigger your symptoms. This may sound easy, but there are several words of caution for this selection process. These caveats include the following:

1. The intermittent nature of IBS symptoms makes it difficult to reproduce the symptoms at all times.

2. The complexity of our everyday diets makes it very difficult to pinpoint offending stimulants. Each meal we eat is made up of multiple foods, and most foods are made up of multiple ingredients.

3. In most cases, a combination of two or more simultaneous triggers provokes the symptoms. Thus, identification of each individual trigger may prove to be very difficult.

Despite these difficulties, this method is still your best option, and you should create a detailed diary of your daily diet and GI symptoms to pinpoint the triggers of your symptoms.

The Dynamic Diet

As you can see, there is no specific diet proven to be effective for IBS. It is important to remember that most individuals react differently to different foods and that symptoms are not always associated with specific foods. Symptoms depend on the dynamic interaction between you, the foods you eat and your environmental stressors. Therefore, we propose a dynamic diet for the management of IBS.

The phrase *dynamic diet* refers to diet modification based on individual experiences. This means that you determine which foods to eat and which foods to exclude, based on your current life situation and your previous experiences. For example, if a specific food makes your GI symptoms worse, you should avoid it. If you do not experience symptoms, you can include that food in your diet.

Foods are divided into three different categories. The first group is comprised of non-stimulant foods. These are the foods you can consume at anytime without experiencing any GI symptoms. The second category, the stimulant group, consists of foods that result in the creation or worsening of symptoms most of the time; these foods should be avoided at all times. The last group consists of those foods that could either be stimulants or non-stimulants based on the situation. Most of these foods will not cause any problem when your disease is not in flare-up phase or when you are not under a lot of environmental stressors; however, they can potentially cause trouble and should be avoided during periods of symptomatic flare-up.

This nutrition workbook is designed to be used as a food diary and will help you to categorize individual food items based on your own experiences. For this reason, it is important to keep a good record of your symptoms and daily diet in order to be able to match this information and create your food list. This should include paying close attention to the types of foods, the ingredients, beverages, and environmental details. You may use the next few pages to create your list, which will be used as the basis for the creation of your dynamic diet.

Classification of Foods

Non-stimulant foods

As mentioned previously, the list of non-stimulant foods should be created by **you**. However, based on information obtained from large surveys of patients, we created a **generic**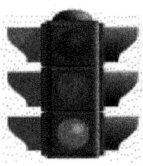

list of non-stimulant foods. This list is generic in the sense that these foods do not cause symptoms for most people who have IBS. It will help you generate ideas for your own list of non-stimulant foods.

Generic Non-Stimulant Foods

Fruits	grapefruit	mangos
	apricots	papayas
	bananas	applesauce
	pears (peeled)	grapes
	apricots (peeled)	raisins
	peaches (peeled)	dates
	nectarines (peeled)	prunes
	apples (peeled)	
Vegetables	potatoes	yams
	chestnuts	squash
	sweet potatos	avocados
	onion (cooked)	pumpkin
	tomatoes (cooked)	rutabagas
	bell peppers (cooked)	parsnips
	cucumbers (peeled/seeded)	lettuce
	eggplant (peeled/seeded)	carrots
	tomatoes (peeled/seeded)	broccoli
Grains	barley	white bread

	lentils corn meal rice flour tortillas	oatmeal quinoa rice cereal pasta
Meats and Protein	lean steamed beef lean baked beef chicken breast without skin turkey breast without skin	soy lean poultry lean fish egg whites
Dairy	lactose-free milk live culture yogurt	skimmed milk
Beverages	warm water apple juice cherry juice green tea	iced tea grape juice carrot juice

Your Non-Stimulant Foods

Use the following table to record your non-stimulant foods.

Fruits	
Vegetables	
Grains	
Meats and Protein	
Dairy	
Beverages	
Other	

Variable foods

The following table contains foods that should be used with caution. Under some circumstances, these foods can cause symptoms. 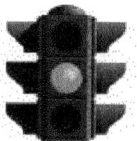 For example, when your IBS is in flare-up or when you are experiencing a period of psychological stress, it may be wise to avoid these groups of foods. As mentioned perviously, you may decide to move a food from this category to either the non-stimulant or the stimulant category, based on your personal experience.

Generic Variable Foods

Fruits	blueberries	blackberries
	strawberries	cranberries
	oranges	grapefruit
	cherries	lemons
	apple (w/skin)	limes
	peaches (w/skin)	pineapple
	nectarines (w/skin)	watermelon
	apricots (w/skin)	other melons
	pears (w/skin)	dried fruit
Vegetables	watercress	fresh herbs
	snow peaks	shallots
	whole peas	leeks
	snap peas	pea pods
	cucumbers	cabbage
	cauliflower	rhubarb
	spinach	collards
	kale	brussels
	uncooked bell peppers	arugula
	fried bell peppers	celery
	uncooked oninon	scallions

	fried oninon	bok choy
	peeled/seeded tomatoes	green beans
	peeled/seeded eggplant	sprouts
	alfalfa	sunflower
	radish	
Grains	gluten	biscuits
	pie crust	wheat
	scones	croissants
	muesli	doughnut
	pastries	granola
Meats and Protein	low fat lean ground beef	shrimp
	breaded patties	scallops
	baked lean beef	soybeans
	Baked lamb	other seafood
	Baked steak	
Beverages	sugar-free juice	lemonade
	Carbonated beverages	Ginger Ale
	Regular Coke	diet Coke
	Regular Pepsi	diet Pepsi
	Sprite	diet Sprite
	root beer	beer
	caffeinated coffee	black tea
	light alcoholic beverages	wine
Dairy	low fat milk	butter
	ice cream	margarine
	plain yogurt	
Other	seeds	popcorn
	french fries	onion rings
	potato chips	nuts
	milk Chocolate	corn chips
	sugars (fructose)	olives
	artificial sweetners (Splenda, sorbitol)	

Your Variable Foods

Use the following table to record your variable foods.

Fruits	
Vegetables	
Grains	
Meat/Protein foods	
Dairy	
Beverages	
Other	

Stimulant foods

Listed below are the foods that may be considered stimulants. For most people with IBS, they are likely to cause symptoms most of the time and should be avoided or used with caution.

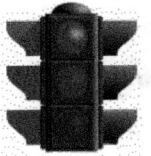

Generic Stimulant Foods

Fruits	pomegranate	Tangerene
Vegetables	jalapeños spicy potato chips turnips	garlic beets
Grains	black pepper other hot spices	red pepper
Meats and Protein	smoked meat deep fried meat marinated meat egg yolks corn dogs nut butters bacon veggie meat substitute veggie burgers regular ground beef roast beef corned beef sausage marbled lamb poultry (dark meat, skin)	fried meat salted meat jerky strips buffalo wings hot dogs shellfish luncheon meat aged steaks pastrami ham marbled beaf marbled pork
Dairy	whole milk cream Cheese cream whipped cream	coconut milk Half-and-Half sour cream Cool Whip
Beverages	Strong alcoholic beverages hi caffein drinks	hard liquor energy drink

18

	espresso flavored soda other carbonated beverages	strong coffee Dr. Pepper
Other	mayonnaise tartar sauce adding extra oil skillet- or pan-fried foods battered and deep-fried foods	salad dressings dark chocolate spreads garlic bread

Your Stimulant Foods

Use the following table to record your stimulant foods.

Fruits	
Vegetables	
Grains	
Meats and Protein	
Dairy	
Beverages	
Other	

Fiber and Your Diet

The addition of fiber to the diet has numerous health benefits.

- ✓ Prevention of coronary heart disease
- ✓ Prevention of colon cancer
- ✓ Regulation of blood sugar
- ✓ Prevention of diverticular disease

Although many of these proclaimed benefits are not well established, there is little doubt that fiber improves bowel movements by increasing the frequency and bulk of the stool and also adds positive bacteria to the colon. Fiber comes from a variety of foods and dietary supplements and is essential to maintaining the health of your gastrointestinal tract. There are two main types of fiber, soluble and insoluble. Solubility refers to how well the fiber dissolves in water and how fermentable it is in the colon. Soluble fiber is highly fermentable by colonic bacteria, whereas insoluble fiber can be fermentable or non-fermentable. Soluble fiber can be viscous, such as oats and legumes, or non-viscous, such as wheat bran and whole grains, whereas all insoluble fibers are non-viscous. The viscosity and the solubility give each fiber its unique characteristics. Generally, the highly fermentable soluble fibers promote lowered cholesterol, addition of beneficial bacteria to the colon, and other significant health effects. Insoluble fiber increases stool bulk, decreases stool transit time, and softens the stool.

Currently it is recommended that persons with IBS increase their **soluble** fiber intake.

Nearly all foods can provide some fiber, with the exception of complete proteins such as meat, poultry, fish, milk, eggs, cheese, butter, and oil. Vegetables, fruits, whole grains, nuts, beans, legumes, and seeds provide the majority of fiber in our diets. Of these foods, most provide both types of fiber, but here are lists of foods that are high in soluble or insoluble fiber.

foods with soluble fiber
oat-based products
barley
peas or pea-starch, beans, lentils, flaxseeds
oranges, grapefruit, citrus fruits, apples, pears, peaches, nectarines, prunes, passion fruit, amaranth, carrots

foods with insoluble fiber
whole wheat, wheat wran
rice bran and brown rice
nuts, seeds, popcorn
fruit skin, berries
vegetables

non-viscous soluble fiber supplements
Benefiber® (wheat dextrin)
short-chain fructooligosaccharides
Nutraflora®
oat bran
Fibersure® (inulin)
FiberChoice®

Additionally, here is a list of supplements that can be used to increase fiber in your diet.

viscous soluble fiber supplements
Metamucil® (psyllium)
Konsyl® (psyllium)
Perdiem®
Fiberall®
Fybogel®
Acacia Tummy Fiber® (acacia gum)
Citrucel® (methylcellulose)
Equalactin® (calcium polycarbophil)
Fibercon

insoluble fiber supplements
wheat bran
raw bran
wheat germ
rice bran

The fiber products available are not limited to the preceding lists. In fact, there are numerous other brand names that provide fiber material and contain one or a mixture of several ingredients mentioned above. This list includes the following:

SteviaPlus Fiber®, Dental Fibers®, Everybody's Fiber®, Fiber Delights®, Fiber Perfect®, Gentle Fibers®, Fiber Force-6®, Multi-Fiber®, Natural Fiber®, Fiber Max®, Daily Fiber®, Chewable Fiber®, Colonix Fiber®, Fiber Plus Caps®, Metamucil Psyllium Fiber Wafers®, Fiber Clean Capsules®, Fiber Fusion®, Everyday Fiber System®, Daily Fiber X®, Daily Fiber®, Activated Fiber Tablets®, Super Fiber Psyllium Seed®, Multi-Fiber Complex®, Daily Fiber

Powder®, Super Seed®, Beyond Fiber®, Thermo-Bond Fiber Tablets®, Brewer's Yeast Plus Fiber®, and Fiber Choice Fiber®.

The recommended intake of fiber is 25 to 35 grams per day or 14 grams per 1000 calories consumed, according to the 2005 Dietary Guidelines for Americans. Side effects of fiber include gas and bloating. To avoid these, it is recommended to start by adding a very small amount of dietary fiber to your diet and to increase the amount slowly. The same is true of fiber supplements which should be started at a small dose (tip of a teaspoon) and gradually increased by 1 to 2 grams every few days, consistently, until you to reach the recommended amount or desired effect. In addition, you may improve the tolerance by using Beano® or simethicone (Gas-X®, Maalox®, Mylanta®) to minimize the side effects of bloating and gas formation. It is recommended to first consider consuming foods that are good sources of natural fiber, rather than supplements, as food provides additional vitamins and minerals that supplements do not.

Furthermore, many fiber supplements have additives, flavorings, colorings, and preservatives. Because some people with IBS are sensitive to these ingredients, you may want to choose a supplement with as few of these additives as possible. In particular, the alcohol sugar sorbitol is found in chewable fiber supplements and should be avoided by people with gastrointestinal issues. You can always seek further advice from your gastroenterologist or registered dietitian regarding your fiber needs and the best way to incorporate fiber into your diet.

Diet and Intestinal Bacteria

Probiotics

There are more than a million species of bacteria in our GI tracts. Probiotics are nutritional supplements that contain beneficial microorganisms or bacteria similar to those found in our GI tract. Probiotics are rapidly becoming a popular and important tool for preserving and maintaining our health. There are currently many different types of probiotics; however, the more common strains are *lactobacillus* and *bifidobacterium*. Evidence suggests that probiotcs may help in treating diarrhea, preventing and treating vaginal yeast infections and urinary tract infections, reducing the recurrence of certain cancers, shortening the duration of intestinal infections, preventing and treating inflammation of the colon after surgery, and, most importantly to us, treating IBS-related symptoms.

Currently, studies on the effectiveness of probiotics in the relief of IBS symptoms have producd varying results. Some studies have observed improvement in flatulence, abdominal pain, transit time, and bacterial counts with the use of probiotics in patients with IBS, while others have found no significant improvement. Results from clinical trials using the specific probiotic VSL#3® have demonstrated a reduction in flatulence and bloating among IBS patients.

While probiotics are not currently considered a standard of practice for the treatment of IBS-related symptoms, there is no evidence to suggest any adverse effects from their use, so probiotics should be strongly considered as a treatment option.

Prebiotics

Prebiotics are non-digestible food that benefits the host by stimulating the growth and/or activity of healthy bacteria in the colon. In order to be considered a prebiotic, the food ingredient must not be broken down or absorbed in the GI tract, is fermented by the GI microflora, and selectively stimulates the growth or activity of intestinal bacteria associated with health and well-being. Prebiotics are found naturally in many foods and can be isolated from plants or synthesized. Traditional sources of prebiotics include soybeans, raw oats, inulin sources, and unrefined wheat and barley.

Since the main characteristic of prebiotics in the diet is to promote the growth and proliferation of beneficial bacteria in the gastrointestinal tract and potentially yield or enhance the effect of probiotic bacteria, it is thought that prebiotics may play a role in improvement in GI health and thus also have an effect on improvement of IBS-related symptoms.

No current well-designed studies exist on prebiotics in IBS. Lactulose, one of the more well-known prebiotics has been successful as treatment for constipation. However, it tends to produce substantial amounts of gas and abdominal pain which may actually aggravate symptoms of IBS. In addition, substances such as oligosaccharides, inulin and galactose may increase stool weight leading to improvement in diarrhea. However, these substances have also been found to increase flatulence and bloating in otherwise healthy individuals, which may be undesirable for patients with IBS.

Given the above, there is no current recommendation for the use of prebiotics in the symptom management of IBS.

Antibiotics

Recently there is a growing concern regarding an imbalance of good and bad bacteria in the gut. Many researchers are using antibiotics to reduce the load of bacteria that are residing in the GI tract. In some studies, a significant number of IBS subjects had abnormal growth of bacteria in the small bowel and responded to a course of antibiotic treatment. Although these results should be confirmed in the future by repeated research, there is no doubt that antibiotics could be helpful in at least a subgroup of patients with IBS. This is particularly true in those with diarrhea-predominant IBS. In this group, further investigation using breath testing or antibiotic trial therapy may be a reasonable approach. The commonly used antibiotics in this setting are those antibiotics that have minimal systemic absorption and will decontaminate the gastrointestinal tract as they travel through it.

Lactose-Free Diet

Lactose, the milk sugar found in certain dairy products, may not be well tolerated in some individuals with IBS. If you feel that you fall into this category, you may want to consider eliminating lactose for two weeks to see if you observe an improvement in symptoms. Sources of lactose include milk, cheese, cottage cheese, ice cream or any food containing dairy as an ingredient such as pasta dishes, pizza, mayonnaise, etc. Yogurt also contains lactose; however, it is still well tolerated because it contains the lactase enzyme produced by the bacterial cultures in the yogurt, which breaks down the lactose. In addition, aged cheese such as cheddar and Parmesan contain less lactose in comparison to fresh cheeses such as Port Salut or mozzarella because the bacteria have had more time to break down the lactose.

If symptoms improve with the elimination of lactose and you choose to continue to exclude it from your diet, it is important to obtain calcium and vitamin D from other food sources. Alternatives to milk include soy milk or rice milk. You may also use an enzyme product such as Lactaid when consuming products with lactose to help with the breakdown.

The Effects of Long Fasting on IBS

Studies on the efficacy of a long period of fasting for IBS are limited. One study from Japan observed symptoms in IBS patients after a 10-day fasting period followed by five days of feeding. Compared with control subjects, researchers found a significant improvement in symptoms with fasting. These findings make sense as symptoms of IBS are typically related to oral intake. Therefore, fasting removes all stimuli from the GI tract that would otherwise cause GI symptoms. Benefit related to a specific length of fasting has not yet been determined. Although, some individuals may experience benefit from the fasting period, others may have an exaggeration of symptoms. Overall, the response of each individual to the fasting period can be quite variable.

Food Allergy vs. IBS

A food allergy is different from IBS because it is an immunological reaction to a particular food or class of foods that usually occurs within two hours of eating a specific allergen. In addition, an allergy causes abdominal pain that is typically accompanied by itching of the lips, inside of the mouth, tongue, or throat and can cause swelling in these areas. Other symptoms such as itchy skin, rash, hives, shortness of breath or even syncope (anaphylactic reaction) may be seen in severe forms of food allergy.

Allergic reaction types and elapsed time to produce a reaction are usually consistent and reproducible, whereas with IBS the reaction may not be consistently produced by the trigger every time. Sometimes the reaction of itching or swelling is only limited to the mouth, known as oral allergy syndrome. The most common food allergies seen in adults are peanuts, tree nuts, fish, shellfish, apples, carrots, bananas, melons, cantaloupe, and tomatoes. Lack of tolerance to milk and dairy products as mentioned above, in most cases, is not due to a milk allergy but instead due to the lack of adequate lactase enzyme in the intestine.

Elimination Diet

In order to determine which ingredient might be the culprit for your symptoms, you may want to try an elimination diet. We recommend starting with foods that have been scientifically proven to have a higher incidence of causing symptoms, such as dairy, gluten, and fructose. In addition, those who have problems mainly due to food allergy may benefit from eliminating the foods that are most likely associated with food allergy such as peanuts, tree nuts, fish, shellfish, apples, carrots, bananas, melons, cantaloupe, and tomatoes. For a description of dairy elimination please refer back to the section on a lactose-free diet.

Some important general rules of the elimination process include:

➢ Eliminate one food from your diet at a time (or one food category at a time, i.e., dairy).

➢ Avoid eating item for a specified amount of time (see next point).

➢ The usual elimination time can be variable based on the type of diet; however, two weeks is a typical period for most food. For gluten, at least a four-week elimination time is suggested.

➢ If no symptoms occur during the elimination process, continue the elimination as this food may be triggering symptoms of IBS.

➤ Many doctors suggest re-introduction of the suspicious food item or food category to prove that it is capable of reproducing the symptoms. Check with your gastroenterologist.

Gluten-free diet

To eliminate gluten from your diet, follow these general recommendations.

➤ Consume whole grain or enriched gluten-free foods (breads, pasta, breakfast cereal).

➤ Consume fresh, frozen, unprocessed, or minimally processed fruits, vegetables, milk products, and protein foods.

➤ Grains and plant foods that can be safely eaten include aramanth, arrowroot, buckwheat, cassava, corn, flax, Indian rice grass, Job's tears, legumes (dry beans, peas, lentils), millet, nuts, potatoes, quinoa, rice, sago, sorghum, soy, tapioca, tef, wild rice, and yucca.

➤ Foods containing the following ingredients should be avoided: wheat (all types including einkorn, emmer, spelt, and kamut), barley, rye, malt and oats (unless gluten free).

For more details on the gluten-free diet or if you have been diagnosed with celiac disease, contact your gastroenterologist or registered dietitian for more comprehensive dietary guidelines.

Fructose-free diet

Fructose is a naturally occurring simple sugar found in fruits, vegetables, and honey. To eliminate fructose from your diet, follow these general recommendations:

➤ Avoid fruits and fruit juices with higher levels of fructose as these may cause gas, bloating, abdominal cramping and diarrhea. Fruits and fruit juices to avoid include prunes, pears, cherries, peaches, apples, plums, applesauce, apple juice, pear juice, apple cider, grapes, and dates.

➤ Eliminate products with ingredients that list fructose, crystalline fructose, honey, and sorbitol on the label.

➤ Avoid sugar alcohols, which include sorbitol, isomalt, lactitol, maltitiol, mannitol, xylitol, erythrytol and lactatol. These are typically found in diet foods such as diet drinks, ice cream, candy, and processed goods.

➤ Limit drinks made with high fructose corn syrup. For example, limit soda intake to 12 ounces per day.

Weekly Menus

Recommended Weekly Menu for Period of IBS Flare-up

Day 1

Breakfast	1/2 cup high-fiber cereal with 1/2 cup fat-free (or soy) milk, 1 banana, 1 cup decaffeinated coffee or tea
Lunch	3 oz water-packed tuna with 1 T light mayonnaise wrapped in whole-wheat flour tortilla, ½ cup carrots
Dinner	6 oz baked chicken, 1 cup whole grain rice, 1 cup steamed broccoli, 1 whole grain roll
Snacks	1 cup unsweetened fruit juice, low-fat yogurt with sliced fruit, 1 oz whole-wheat crackers

Day 2

Breakfast	3 scrambled egg whites, 1/2 chopped bell pepper, 1/2 cup fat-free milk
Lunch	6″ whole-wheat tortilla, 3 oz low-fat sliced turkey, 1/2 avocado
Dinner	4 oz grilled fish, 1/2 cup spinach, 2 slices French bread
Snacks	1/2 cup sorbet, 1 mango, 2 oz rye crackers

Day 3

Breakfast	1 cup soy yogurt, 2 T sugar-free granola, 1 peeled apple, 1 cup decaffeinated coffee or tea
Lunch	1 cup lentil soup, 1 whole-wheat pita, 2 cups mixed salad leaves, 2 T fat-free dressing
Dinner	3 oz grilled low-fat pork tenderloin, 1/2 cup pasta, 1/2 cup applesauce, 1 whole-grain dinner roll
Snacks	1 slice oat bread with light margarine, 1 banana, 2 hard boiled egg whites

Day 4

Breakfast	1 cup oatmeal, 1/2 cup fat-free milk, 1 cup berries
Lunch	1 open-face tuna melt with 3 oz tuna and 1 slice low-fat cheddar cheese, 1 cup unsweetened fruit juice
Dinner	1 cup cooked pasta, 3 turkey meatballs, 2 oz marinara sauce, 1/2 cup steamed broccoli
Snacks	1/2 cup mango juice, 1 oz whole-wheat crackers, 1/2 cup baby carrots

Day 5

Breakfast	1/2 cup high fiber cereal with 1/2 cup soy milk, 1/2 grapefruit
Lunch	1 whole-wheat pita with 4 oz turkey breast, 1 cup sliced bell peppers, 2 tsp olive oil, 1 cup spinach
Dinner	3 turkey tacos made with ground turkey and whole-wheat tortillas, 1/2 cup brown rice
Snacks	1 cup yogurt, 1 peeled apple, 1 oz low-fat cheese

Day 6

Breakfast	3 scrambled egg whites with 1/2 cup spinach, 1/2 cup fat-free milk
Lunch	2 slices rye bread with 1 T light mayonnaise and 1/2 sliced fresh tomato and 1/2 sliced avocado
Dinner	4 oz lean grilled chicken breast with lemon juice and pepper, 1 cup salad greens, 1/2 boiled potato
Snacks	1 whole-wheat pita bread with 1 oz hummus, 1 cup unsweetened fruit juice

Day 7

Breakfast	1 cup soy yogurt parfait with 1/2 cup berries and 2 T low-fat granola
Lunch	1 whole-wheat tortilla with 3 oz sliced chicken breast, mixed greens, tomato slices, 1/2 grapefruit
Dinner	4 oz grilled lean fish, 1/2 cup brown rice, 1 cup salad greens
Snacks	1 cup sorbet, 1 banana, 1/2 whole-wheat pita bread

Your Weekly Menu for Period of IBS Flare-up

Day 1

Breakfast	
Lunch	
Dinner	
Snacks	

Day 2

Breakfast	
Lunch	
Dinner	
Snacks	

Day 3

Breakfast	
Lunch	
Dinner	
Snacks	

Day 4

Breakfast	
Lunch	
Dinner	
Snacks	

Day 5

Breakfast	
Lunch	
Dinner	
Snacks	

Day 6

Breakfast	
Lunch	
Dinner	
Snacks	

Day 7

Breakfast	
Lunch	
Dinner	
Snacks	

This handout and workbook is designed to improve your overall knowledge about various aspects of your diet and to help you explore your dietary choices to build a diet that best suits your condition. This commonsense approach could be one of the most useful and least restrictive diet modifications you may select to manage your IBS.

Please take the time to register on our website at http://www.IHaveIBS.com to receive our complementary monthly newsletter, IBS*Times*. This will help keep you up to date on the latest developments and research in the field of irritable bowel syndrome and its management.

If you have any more questions regarding your diet that you can not find in this book, you may ask your question on the website http://www.IHaveIBS.com. We will be more than happy to answer your questions and also potentially post these questions, excluding your personal information, in our monthly newsletter, IBS*Times*.

www.ingramcontent.com/pod-product-compliance
Lightning Source LLC
Chambersburg PA
CBHW070842310526
45793CB00011B/514